NATURE'S ALTERNATIVE TO ANTIBIOTICS

Viruses and bacteria are scary because most of them are invisible to the naked eye. Our fight against these unseen enemies has been incredibly successful thanks to the development of bacteria-killing antibiotics during World War II. Since then antibiotics have been prescribed for every type of infection from tuberculosis to the common cold, making them the most popular drugs in history. This overreliance on—and sometimes unthinking overuse of—antibiotics in the past fifty years has made nearly every disease-causing bacterium stronger and more resistant to drugs. "Controlled" diseases such as tuberculosis, pneumonia and typhoid have come back to life. Even head lice and scabies, parasites once equated with the poor and malnourished, are taking up residence in the well-to-do.

As medical researchers look for answers to these vexing problems, a growing number of people are turning away from conventional medicine's reliance on synthetic drugs and magic bullets and are rediscovering tea tree oil and grapefruit seed extract, two powerful yet natural antiseptics. Tea tree oil and grapefruit seed extract are entirely different substances; they come from very different plants and are extracted in different ways, yet as you'll find out in the pages that follow, their uses and results are startlingly similar and effective.

ABOUT THE AUTHOR

CJ Puotinen has studied with some of America's leading herbalists and is a member of the Herb Research Foundation, the American Herb Association, the International Herb Association and the Northeast Herbal Association. In addition to magazine and journal articles on health and medicinal herbs, she is the author of *Herbal Teas, Herbs to Help You Breathe Freely, Herbs for Men's Health, Herbs for Arthritis* and *Herbs to Improve Digestion,* all published by Keats Publishing, Inc.

Nature's Antiseptics
Tea Tree Oil and Grapefruit Seed Extract

Using them to treat 30 health
problems, from abrasions to warts

CJ Puotinen

Keats Publishing, Inc. 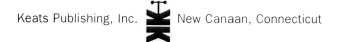 New Canaan, Connecticut

Nature's Antiseptics: Tea Tree Oil and Grapefruit Seed Extract is not intended as medical advice. Its intent is solely informational and educational. Please consult a health professional should the need for one be indicated.

NATURE'S ANTISEPTICS: TEA TREE OIL AND GRAPEFRUIT SEED EXTRACT

ISBN: 0-87983-714-4

Printed in the United States of America

8 9 10 DIG/DIG 12

Contents

	Page
Introduction	6
Australian Tea Tree Oil	9
Grapefruit Seed Extract	12
Making Your Own Antiseptics	15
Using Nature's Two Best Germ-Fighters to Treat Over 30 Common Conditions	19
Improving on Personal Care Products	44
Resources	46
Bibliography	48

INTRODUCTION

The germ theory of disease is alive and well in the United States. Our household cleansers contain disinfecting bleach; our best-selling hand and body soaps kill germs of every description. Since they were developed during World War II, bacteria-killing antibiotics have been prescribed for every type of infection, making them the most popular drugs in history. In our scariest TV commercials, germs collect in kitchen drains, toilet bowls, bathtubs, shower stalls, kitchen counters and telephones, waiting to infect us all. More frightening than germs at home are the microbes that lurk in public water supplies, hospitals, restaurants and even in the open air. Every year more of us buy water filters, bottled water, germicidal sprays and other protection. Fear of food poisoning has changed our cooking habits. Gone are the days of raw eggs and rare meat, especially hamburger; now warning labels on beef and poultry remind supermarket customers to serve everything well done. We peel our apples and scrub our vegetables, sometimes in disinfecting chemicals. Japan may surpass us in the germ phobia department—people there wear surgical masks when they have a cold—but we run a close second. Pathogens are our enemy.

From time to time, events prove us right. When cryptosporidium, *Giardia lamblia* and other microbes contaminate our water supplies, hundreds fall ill. In only fifty years of use, antibiotics like penicillin have made nearly every disease-causing bacterium stronger and more resistant to drugs, so that illnesses like tuberculosis, pneumonia and typhoid, recently considered extinct, are once again fatal. When several children died in Washington State in 1993, the killer was a bacterium, *E. coli* 0157:H7, in undercooked hamburgers from a fast food restaurant. Salmonella and botulism make headlines every year. So do unusual infections like Legionnaire's disease, which contaminates the air ducts of some hotels and cruise ships. Reports of an Ebola virus outbreak in Africa, followed by a dramatic book and movie, give us nightmares. Closer to home, the Hanta virus strikes without warning. Health experts warn that we are overdue for a worldwide flu epidemic like the famous flu pandemic of 1918, which killed millions, including my husband's grandfather and probably some relatives of yours as well. Viruses and bacteria are scary because they're invisible to the naked eye, but not all our enemies are microscopic. Tapeworms, hookworms, roundworms, threadworms, pinworms and other parasites once equated with the poor, ignorant and malnourished have taken up residence in the well-to-do. Even head lice and scabies are making a comeback.

As medical researchers look for answers to these vexing problems, a growing number of Americans are turning away from conventional medicine's reliance on synthetic drugs and magic bullets. Experts from the American Society of Microbiology (ASM) issued an unusual public warning in 1995, stating that our overreliance on antibiotic drugs has created a serious and imminent danger. "There is little doubt that the problem [of drug-resistant bacteria] is global in scope and very serious," they stated. The cause is the unthinking overuse of antibiotics over several decades, including prescriptions for penicillin and similar drugs in the treatment of illnesses they have no effect on, like the common cold. Hospitals are especially efficient at breeding drug-resistant bacteria, for they collect people with impaired immune systems and give them heavy doses of powerful antibiotics. Any bacteria that mutate and survive have an excellent chance of spreading to impaired immune systems nearby. These conditions have brought tuberculosis, pneumonia and other "controlled" diseases back to life. While acknowledging that exotic viruses like Ebola are a serious matter, the ASM experts concluded, "We are in greater danger from common disease-producing organisms that are becoming increasingly resistant to antibiotics than from any exotic outbreak in the hot zone."

The bleach industry wants you to know that inexpensive

chlorine laundry bleach kills just about everything: molds, bacteria, even the Ebola virus. For years the U.S. government has recommended that foreign service employees living in developing nations disinfect their fruits, vegetables, meat, fish, eggs and chicken in dilute solutions of bleach and water. Bleach can also be used on cutting surfaces, knives, refrigerator handles, cupboard doors and floors to eliminate pathogens. Considering that most cases of food poisoning are believed to originate in private homes due to the careless handling of raw meat and poultry, disinfecting kitchen surfaces is a sensible precaution.

But chlorine bleach has side effects. It can ruin clothes, contribute to respiratory problems and, if accidentally mixed with ammonia, actually poison you with chlorine gas. Doctors who treat environmental illnesses consider chlorine a toxin we should all avoid, claiming that it increases the risk of bladder, breast, larynx and rectal cancers and may play a role in heart disease. As swimmers know, chlorine can cause skin irritations and leave you with red, burning eyes.

Wouldn't it be nice if there were a nontoxic disinfectant, something that would work as well as chlorine and other chemical antiseptics yet not pose a hazard to our clothes or our health? Wouldn't it be nice if that product could treat our bodies as well as our homes, making us less hospitable hosts to the viruses, bacteria, molds, yeasts and parasites that want to live in us? And wouldn't it be nice if such a product were inexpensive and easy to find?

Yes it would, and the best part of this story is that nature has blessed us with not one but two such antiseptics. Tea tree oil and grapefruit seed extract are entirely different substances; they come from very different plants and are extracted in different ways, yet their uses and results are startlingly similar.

AUSTRALIAN TEA TREE OIL

In the summer of 1984, my husband and I vacationed along the cool, green Oregon coast. Nearly every tiny town seemed to have at least one shop advertising on a large sign, "Nail fungus? We have Melaleuca!"

We finally stopped to satisfy our curiosity. *Melaleuca*, we were told, is a magical oil from Australia that has all kinds of uses, including the treatment of toenail fungi so common in damp climates. The man who sold us our first bottle of what is now more commonly called tea tree oil listed a dozen conditions it was guaranteed to correct. When my husband asked about athlete's foot, our salesman said that when he began using tea tree oil shampoo every morning in the shower, his athlete's foot disappeared along with his dandruff. Cuts, infected wounds, burns, acne, head colds, jock itch, ringworm, strained muscles—there seemed no end to the conditions this essential oil could improve.

Melaleuca alternifolia is one of over 300 varieties of tea tree or *Melaleuca* and apparently the only one with medicinal properties. And not all *Melaleuca alternifolia* are alike; the most medicinal oil comes from trees growing in a tiny section of New South Wales, Australia. Trees growing elsewhere produce inferior oils.

The Australian tea tree got its name in 1770 from Captain Cook, whose crew, while exploring the countryside, discovered that its aromatic leaves made a spicy tea. Aborigines living around Bungawalbyn Creek, the area known for superior tea trees, treated cuts, wounds and skin infections with crushed leaves and warm mud. When white loggers arrived in search of tall cedar, and later when settlers cleared the land for farming, they were introduced to the plant's healing properties. The tea tree has a long history of therapeutic use.

In the early 1920s an Australian chemist, Dr. A. Penfold, tested the tree's essential oil and found its antiseptic powers to be 13 times stronger than carbolic acid, then the standard for disinfectants. Penfold's findings, presented to the Royal Society of New South Wales and England, were followed by decades of medical research papers demonstrating the oil's effectiveness in treating skin fungus, gum disease, gynecological infections, athlete's foot, sore throats and nail fungus.

The Medical Journal of Australia published an article titled "A New Australian Germicide" in 1930, reporting that tea tree oil effectively treated septic wounds, carbuncles and pus-filled infections. "The results obtained in a variety of conditions when it was first tried were most encouraging," the report stated, "a striking feature being that it dissolved the pus and left the surface of infected wounds clean, so that its germicidal action became more effective without any apparent damage to the tissues. This was something new, as most efficient germicides destroy tissue as well as bacteria." Tea tree oil's antiseptic properties and its lack of toxic, irritating ingredients made it unique.

After World War II, when antibiotics took the world by storm, natural remedies like tea tree oil fell from favor. It wasn't until the public began to be aware of the dangers of toxic substances and synthetic drugs that tea tree oil was rediscovered. Most of the credit for its commercial success goes to Christopher Dean, whose stepfather, Eric White, planted the world's first tea tree farm, Thursday Plantation, in New South Wales. The plantation produced a high quality oil that Dean and his wife marketed as "a medicine kit in a bottle." The rest, as they say, is history.

The thin, clear, colorless oil has a distinctive aroma and a pungent taste. It reminds many people of turpentine or eucalyptus oil, and while some find the scent and taste objectionable, most come to enjoy it. A complex substance, tea tree oil contains 48 organic compounds, including terpinenes, cymones, pinenes, terpineols, cineole, sesquiterpenes, sesquiterpinene alcohols, veridiflorene, L-terpineol and ally-hexanoate, some of which are found nowhere else in nature. Researchers believe it is the combined effect of these compounds, not the presence of a single substance, that makes the oil so versatile and effective. Its complexity is given credit for tea tree oil's consistent destruction of harmful viruses and bacteria, even after repeated exposure. Some medical researchers believe that the reason so many bacteria have become resistant to antibiotics is that synthetic drugs have a simple structure, making it easy for pathogens to mutate and adapt to their presence. Complex compounds are far more difficult for pathogens to deal with.

Tea trees from the north coast of New South Wales produce a superior oil containing a high percentage of medicinal terpenes and a low percentage of cineole. Cineole gives off a camphorlike odor and is itself medicinal, especially in relieving colds, but it irritates the skin and mucous membranes. Oils containing a high concentration of cineole are too caustic and those with a low concentration of terpenes are less effective. The Australian government helped stabilize tea tree oil products when it required that Oil of Melaleuca contain at least 30 percent terpinen-4-ol, which has been identified as the oil's major germicidal component, and at most 15 percent cineole. Trees producing the highest quality oil generate over 45 percent terpinen-4-ol and less than 3 percent cineole. Because terpinen-4-ol and cineole concentrations vary, so do individual reactions to the resulting oils. If a full-strength tea tree oil causes skin irritation, try another brand.

Those with sensitive skin are encouraged to test tea tree oil by applying a small amount to the inner arm. Any allergic reaction or irritation will manifest within a few minutes. Dilute tea tree oil in an equal quantity of carrier oil or mix it with alcohol and water before trying another patch test. Allergic reactions to tea tree oil are unusual; reactions to diluted tea tree oil are rare.

Note: Never use full-strength tea tree oil on infants, children or pets; always dilute it first. Keep tea tree oil away from the eyes. In case of eye contact, rinse thoroughly with cold water. In case of accidental ingestion, do not induce vomiting. Drink large amounts of water, and, if available, take activated charcoal tablets to absorb the oil within the stomach.

Tea tree oil is considered very safe when used in minute

quantities in the mouth as a treatment for gum disease or canker sores, in the throat as a gargle, or in toothpastes and mouthwashes.

One of the claims made for tea tree oil is that a 15 percent solution is as effective as full-strength oil in killing yeast cells, mold, bacteria and viruses. This was demonstrated in research reported in the U.S. *Journal of the National Medical Association* and the *British Medical Journal* in the 1930s. Full-strength tea tree oil, then called Ti-trol, and a 15 percent solution of tea tree oil, then called Melasol, were tested by dentists for pyorrhea, gingivitis, nerve-capping and hemorrhages, and by doctors for throat infections, gynecological conditions, pus-filled infections and skin fungi, all with excellent results. A 1936 report published by Australian Essential Oils summarized these medical discoveries and noted that doctors and dentists observed that while Ti-trol, the pure oil, had greater penetration through unbroken skin, Melasol, the dilute solution, was more effective in treating infected cuts. The dilute solution mixed more readily with broken tissue, pus and membranes. Subsequent laboratory tests have shown that concentrations as low as 1 percent are effective against streptococcus and other gram-positive bacteria, *E. coli* and other gram-negative bacteria and several fungi.

GRAPEFRUIT SEED EXTRACT

In the 1970s an immunologist, Dr. Jacob Harich, searched for a natural alternative to antibiotics, a nontoxic substance that would help the human body resist bacteria, viruses, parasites and fungi. He found it in the seeds and connecting tissue of grapefruit.

Because of its ability to kill germs on contact, grapefruit seed extract was first adopted by the cosmetic industry, which used it as a preservative. In the food transport business, it provided an alternative to chemicals and irradiation in the shipping of fish, grapes and poultry; grapefruit seed extract is now used to preserve a variety of fruits and vegetables.

Holistic physicians experimenting with grapefruit seed extract, which is safe for internal use, found it effective in treating staphylococcus, streptococcus, salmonella, *Amoeba histolytica* and other parasites, viruses, *Candida albicans*, herpes, sore throats, ear infections, gum disease, athlete's foot, nail fungus and traveler's diarrhea.

According to Dr. Allan Sachs, a spokesman for grapefruit seed extract manufacturers, "Many prestigious universities and independent laboratories have tested grapefruit seed extract against more than 30 fungi, 20 bacteria and a host of viruses and protozoa. In almost all of these cultures grapefruit seed extract exhibited significant antimicrobial activity at low concentration. The famous Pasteur Institute in France, Europe's leading AIDS research institute, has been actively studying the possible application of grapefruit seed extract in AIDS prevention."

Unlike tea tree oil, grapefruit seed extract can be taken internally in therapeutic doses with no adverse side effects. However, some health care professionals believe that the long-term daily use of grapefruit seed extract may disrupt the balance of intestinal flora and suggest alternating grapefruit seed extract with other herbs or supplements for prolonged use. For self-care, consider limiting courses of treatment to four to six weeks and consult an experienced health care practitioner before taking the product for longer periods.

The liquid extract has a bitter, unpleasant taste, but manufacturers now offer a debittered powder in capsules. Campers report that by adding enough liquid extract to taste, they successfully disinfect water on the trail. The bitter taste is, if anything, reassuring. Considering that nearly every lake in North America carries *Giardia lamblia*, a microscopic parasite that causes intestinal disease, a tiny bottle of grapefruit seed extract can make any camping or hiking trip more pleasant. Grapefruit seed extract performs well in very dilute concentrations in a range of 1 part in 200 to 1 part in 50,000.

Because grapefruit seed extract is so new on the holistic health scene, it hasn't enjoyed the decades of medical research and journal reports that have documented the growth of the tea tree oil industry. Holistic health practitioners are just beginning to use grapefruit seed extract as a natural antibiotic, immune system booster, Candida treatment and parasite therapy. Some theorize that its antimicrobial activity enhances the action of herbs such as goldenseal and echinacea, which are often used to prevent or cure colds, flu and other diseases. Grapefruit seed extract has also been used in combination with astragalus, barberry, white oak bark, witch hazel, calendula, slippery elm bark, pau d'arco bark, castor bean extract, artemisia, milk thistle seed, dandelion, plantain and others. The extract may augment the healing activity of these plants.

Grapefruit seed extract is also called grapefruit extract and citrus seed extract. The liquid extract is very concentrated and should be used carefully. Externally, grapefruit seed extract can be diluted with water and used as a facial cleanser. It can be applied full strength to fingernails or toenails to combat fungal infections. A few drops added to shampoo or hair conditioner make an effective scalp treatment that helps control dandruff. A few drops diluted in oil or water treat ear infections. Several drops taken in juice or water help prevent diarrhea, traveler's diarrhea, parasites and viral infections. Mixed with water it makes an effective mouthwash or throat gargle. One drop added to 2 ounces water can be used as a nasal rinse. Several drops in a sink of cold water will disinfect fruits, vegetables, meat, fish, eggs or chicken. Dilute solutions of grapefruit seed extract disinfect toothbrushes, humidifiers, vaporizers, Water Pik units and similar appliances.

A capsule of powdered, debittered extract can be opened so the powdered extract can be sprinkled on food or mixed with water for disinfecting. One capsule is equivalent to approximately 10 to 15 drops of liquid extract and can be used for the same purposes.

A WEALTH OF NEW PRODUCTS

Full-strength tea tree oil and grapefruit seed extract have been called "a medicine kit in a bottle" and "the Swiss Army knife of germ control." Both disinfect whatever they touch when used full strength or in dilute solutions. Both have numerous external applications, many of them overlapping, and grapefruit seed extract can be used internally as well. Products containing these natural antiseptics are still being developed.

Many health food stores now carry tea tree oil soaps, shampoos, toothpaste, dental floss, mouthwash, skin cleansers, bubble baths, massage oils, lip balms, ointments, lozenges for sore throats and special products for pets. Tea tree oil has been added to foot and body powders, laundry detergents, kitchen cleansers and disinfecting air sprays.

Grapefruit seed extract is sold as a liquid concentrate, and in capsules, ear drops, gum cleansers, foot powders, herbal cleansing sprays, feminine rinses, nail treatments, skin cleansers, dental gels, shower gels and bath products.

MAKING YOUR OWN ANTISEPTICS

TEA TREE OIL

Tea tree oil does not dissolve in water. If you add five drops to an ounce of water and shake well, the oil will float to the surface and stay there. Most books and articles about tea tree oil recommend using tea tree oil in this way (adding a measured amount to bath water, vaginal douches, foot soaks, mouthwashes and the like) but even if you shake the liquid vigorously, the distribution of oil will be uneven.

Whenever you prefer to use a dilute solution rather than

full-strength tea tree oil, take an intermediate step and prepare a water-soluble tea tree oil concentrate. This concentrate is very versatile: it can be used in the same way full-strength oil is used, or it can be diluted with large or small amounts of water, herbal tea or aloe vera gel.

WATER-SOLUBLE TEA TREE OIL CONCENTRATE

Here are three ways to make a water-soluble concentrate, using isopropyl (rubbing) alcohol, grain alcohol or vegetable glycerine. If your goal is to make a lotion that will treat athlete's foot, jock itch, cuts, burns and other skin conditions, use isopropyl alcohol and label the container for external use only. Isopropyl alcohol is toxic and should never be swallowed. To make a mouthwash for treating thrush or gum disease, use grain alcohol or vegetable glycerine.

The following are general guidelines and you are encouraged to experiment. Tea tree oil dissolves readily in small amounts of isopropyl alcohol. You will need larger amounts of grain alcohol to dissolve the same amount of tea tree oil, and results will vary depending on the alcohol's proof and other factors.

Have on hand a small, clear glass jar with a tight-fitting lid or a transparent plastic bottle. Combine the tea tree oil and alcohol or glycerine in the jar, close the lid tightly and shake vigorously. Let the jar stand for a minute. Do drops of oil rise to the surface? Does a thin film rise? Or is the liquid uniformly cloudy? If any oil rises to the surface, add more alcohol or glycerine until all the oil has dissolved.

Keep this solution in a container labeled *Water-Soluble Tea Tree Oil Concentrate,* or dilute it with water, herbal tea or aloe vera gel or juice for use as a mouthwash, body wash, foot treatment, pet spray, vaginal douche, sunburn treatment or other purpose. Label the result so you remember what it contains, especially if you used isopropyl alcohol, which should be labeled for external use only.

The following proportions have worked well for me. Adjust them as needed.

1. Mix 1 ounce (2 tablespoons) full-strength tea tree oil and ½ ounce (1 tablespoon) isopropyl rubbing alcohol.

Shake well. If oil floats to the surface, add more alcohol and shake again. Label for external use only.

2. If you can purchase high-proof grain alcohol in your state, try to find 192-proof Everclear or a similar brand of neutral grain spirits. Next best is 151-proof rum. The higher the proof, the higher the alcohol content. You can use any distilled spirit for this purpose—gin, brandy, rum, whatever—but most herbalists and aromatherapists prefer to use vodka or neutral grain spirits because they are fragrance free. Eighty-proof alcohol, widely sold in America, is only 40 percent alcohol and 60 percent water, so you will need more of it to dissolve the oil.

Start with 1 ounce (2 tablespoons) full-strength tea tree oil and add an equal amount of 192-proof Everclear alcohol, 3 tablespoons 151-proof rum or 6 tablespoons 80-proof alcohol. Shake well. If oil floats to the surface, add more alcohol and shake again. When the liquid is uniformly cloudy and no oily film floats to the surface, you have a true solution. Note that a solution made from 80-proof vodka will be less concentrated because of its higher water content than one made with 192-proof Everclear.

3. Glycerine made from cattle bones is sold in drug stores, but most herbalists prefer to use vegetable glycerine, which is sold in health food stores and herbal supply shops. Glycerine's sweet taste makes it a popular solvent in tincture making, especially when alcohol is not appropriate, such as when making tinctures for children. Vegetable glycerine will add a sweet taste to your tea tree oil mouthwash and it adds a soft, emollient touch to skin lotions and after-shave lotions.

Combine 1 ounce (2 tablespoons) full-strength tea tree oil and 2 ounces (4 tablespoons) vegetable glycerine. Add 1 ounce (2 tablespoons) water and shake well. If any oil rises to the surface, add more glycerine and shake again.

Note that these same procedures work with any essential oil, not just tea tree oil. Water-soluble solutions of essential oils can be the foundation of many aromatherapy products, from bath lotions to air sprays.

THE 15 PERCENT SOLUTION

A solution of 15 percent tea tree oil has been shown to be as effective, in most cases, as full-strength tea tree oil. To make a 15 percent solution, take any of the above water-soluble tea tree oil concentrates, each of which contains 1 ounce of full-strength tea tree oil, and add enough water, herbal tea, aloe vera gel or any combination of these to make 6 ounces (¾ cup) solution.

This 15 percent solution can be applied externally, used on infants and pets and, if made with grain alcohol or glycerine, used to treat mouth and gum conditions. Any of these antiseptic solutions can be sprayed on kitchen and bathroom surfaces, in air ducts and air conditioning units, on telephone receivers and mildewed shower walls, added to laundry wash water or simply sprayed into the air.

OIL SOLUTIONS

Water isn't the only way to dilute tea tree oil. Sometimes an oil solution is more appropriate. Massage oils containing tea tree oil treat tired, aching muscles, foot oils cure athlete's foot and hot oil treatments for the hair and scalp are both a beauty treatment and dandruff therapy.

To dilute tea tree oil in a carrier oil such as olive oil, add 1 ounce (2 tablespoons) full-strength tea tree oil to 4 ounces (½ cup) or more of the carrier oil, depending on the oil's purpose and your personal preference. One ounce of tea tree oil in 4 ounces carrier oil produces a 20 percent concentration of tea tree oil. To treat a fungus condition like athlete's foot, this is probably the concentration you will want to try first; for an all purpose massage oil with mild antiseptic properties, use a larger quantity of carrier oil.

Tea tree oil will remain fresh for long periods, more than ten years, if stored in fully filled, well-sealed glass bottles away from heat and light. High-grade plastics can be used for dilute solutions, shampoos, mouthwashes and similar products, but glass containers are recommended for full-strength oil.

DILUTING GRAPEFRUIT SEED EXTRACT

Liquid grapefruit seed extract, which contains vegetable glycerine, is already water soluble, so it can be added to any liquid and will dissolve. The usual recommendation is to add 20 to 40 drops of concentrate to a load of laundry, bathtub, bucket of floor wash water, automatic dishwasher or sink full of dishes. Add 3 to 4 drops to a Water Pik reservoir and slightly more to a humidifier, dehumidifier or vaporizer. Use similar amounts of water-soluble tea tree oil concentrate. There are no hard and fast rules. Both products are forgiving and flexible; use common sense and experiment.

USING NATURE'S TWO BEST GERM FIGHTERS TO TREAT OVER 30 COMMON CONDITIONS

ABRASIONS

Remember skinning your knee on gravel or concrete when you were a child? The resulting scrape is an abrasion, an area of scratched, sore skin that, left unprotected, can become infected and even more painful. Bruising often accompanies abrasions, and the scraped area can be sensitive to heat and pressure.

To prevent an abrasion from becoming infected, paint its surface with full-strength or diluted tea tree oil or grapefruit seed extract. Bandage lightly, if at all. As scabbing occurs and healing skin grows taut over the area, keep it lubricated and flexible with a healing salve or oil, such as vitamin E oil from a supplement capsule. Vitamin E oil mixes readily with both tea tree oil and grapefruit seed extract; the combination speeds healing and helps prevent scarring.

ABSCESSES, BOILS, CARBUNCLES

Abscesses form when pus accumulates somewhere in the body. The infected area, which may be internal or external, swells and becomes inflamed and tender. The infection may be accompanied by alternating chills and fever. Some require surgery, but most are treated with antibiotics.

Boils (also called furuncles) are round, inflamed, tender, itching pus-filled skin infections caused by bacteria, allergies, dietary imbalances, infected wounds or the infection of a hair follicle. A boil becomes a carbuncle when infection spreads, forming additional boils. These skin inflammations appear suddenly, becoming red and swollen within a single day, most often on the scalp, face, neck, underarms or buttocks. Boils usually heal by themselves within two to three weeks, and doctors often drain very large boils.

To treat abscesses, boils or carbuncles at home, apply moist heat several times a day by placing a warm washcloth on the infected area. For best results, soak the cloth in a hot solution of Epsom salts or sea salt, wring out and let cool slightly, then apply as a compress. Hold the compress in place for 10 minutes or longer, with a thick towel over it to retain heat.

Take warm Epsom salt baths for abscesses or boils on the body and add a tablespoon of water-soluble tea tree oil concentrate or grapefruit seed extract to the bath water. Soak for at least 15 minutes. After each treatment, apply full-strength or diluted tea tree oil or diluted grapefruit seed extract. Both disinfectants prevent the spread of infection by killing staphylococcus bacteria. Tea tree oil is said to have a special affinity for pus-filled infections, so its application should speed healing. Some health practitioners have found that honey applied directly to a boil is efficacious; add a few drops of tea tree oil to a tablespoon of honey for an even more effective poultice.

ACNE

Nearly every teenager has some experience with acne, the unsightly skin eruptions that infect the sebaceous glands.

No one knows the exact cause of blackheads, whiteheads or pimples, but most dermatologists believe that diet, heredity, oily skin and hormones play a role. There isn't much one can do about the last three factors, but diets can be changed. Acne is far less common in populations that consume little or no animal fat. The most lasting way to improve facial skin is to increase one's consumption of raw fruits and vegetables and avoid dairy products, chocolate, fatty meats, deep-fried anything, sugar, alcohol and caffeine.

Externally, keep your skin clean but avoid harsh, abrasive soaps or scrubs. Shampoo hair frequently, as oily hair can exacerbate the condition. Add a few drops of tea tree oil or grapefruit seed extract to shampoos, conditioners and face soap. Apply diluted tea tree oil or diluted grapefruit seed extract to your skin as a wash or final rinse, and apply full-strength tea tree oil with a Q-tip or similar cotton swab to trouble spots three or more times daily, as needed.

ARTHRITIS

Arthritis is the painful inflammation of joints such as the knees, fingers, toes, elbows, hips or shoulders, sometimes accompanied by a sharp, grinding pain or by a dull, continuing ache. The most common forms of this disease are osteoarthritis and rheumatoid arthritis. Although most physicians scoff at the notion that food sensitivities may cause arthritis, some patients have documented a connection. By eating dairy products for a week, for example, I can generate painful arthritis in my hands and shoulders; by avoiding milk, yogurt, cheese, cream and other milk-based foods, I stay symptom free. Some people are sensitive to members of the nightshade family, which include eggplants, potatoes, tomatoes, red or green peppers and tobacco.

Because exercise is so important to arthritis sufferers, and because their illness makes exercise so painful, many analgesic rubs and massage oils have been developed over the centuries to alleviate discomfort and restore mobility. Often these creams and lotions change the skin's sensation of temperature, cooling it with mint or warming it with cayenne pepper. Tea tree oil has a slightly cooling effect when applied full strength, in a dilute solution or in a massage oil, but it quickly warms and gradually improves mobility while decreasing pain. Just about every book, pamphlet or brochure describing tea tree oil has an arthritis success story to report. Most suggest adding 3 to 5 drops of tea tree oil to a small amount of baby oil or massage oil, then rubbing it into inflamed joints. Repeat twice daily and use for several days, then use as needed.

BRUISES

When bruised, the skin remains unbroken but its underlying tissues are damaged, painful and swollen. Black-and-blue marks are caused by blood collecting under the skin in response to hitting a hard object. The herb most associated with bruise repair is arnica (*Arnica montana* and other species) because alcohol tinctures, salves and massage oils made from its yellow blossoms stimulate and dilate the capillaries, increasing the exchange of blood at the injury site.

Tea tree oil has a similar effect and, in addition, it has analgesic properties. Because it penetrates quickly through the skin to the injury, it helps begin repair work at once, and it alleviates pain at the same time. My favorite bruise therapy is 4 parts arnica tincture combined with 1 part tea tree oil applied every few hours for two or three days, as needed. If applied within a few minutes of injury, this combination truly stops pain, swelling and bruising on contact; applied after bruising develops, it reduces pain and speeds healing. If desired, follow with an ice pack or cold compress.

BURNS

The first thing to do in case of a burn is cool the skin. Immerse the burned area in cold water until all heat from the burn dissipates and pain begins to subside, usually within ten minutes for minor burns. If you have full-strength tea tree oil on hand, apply it even before you submerge the injury, for tea tree oil does not dissolve in water and it will remain in place as the burn cools. Do not try to remove clothing that may be stuck to the burn, but cut away what you can. Obviously, if the burn is serious you should seek medical attention.

A little-known treatment for burns, even serious burns, is honey. As beekeeper Ross Conrad reported in a 1993 edition of the *Northeast Herbal Association Journal*, raw honey has a long history of use in the treatment of burns. When serious burns are treated conventionally, dressing changes are extremely painful, but when honey is the only dressing, burns heal quickly and dressing changes are painless and require no scraping. Coating a burn with honey retards oxygenation by sealing the wound, which alleviates pain within seconds. Honey is hydroscopic, absorbing moisture from its surroundings, so it doesn't dry out and its pH is too acid for bacterial growth. Dr. Dennis Cavanagh, Chairman of the Department of Gynecology and Obstetrics at St. Louis University School of Medicine, used honey to accelerate the healing of surgical wounds, all of which responded promptly in his clinical trial. "Wounds were bacteriologically sterile within three to six days," Cavanagh reported, "and remained so until completely united. . . . Honey is much more efficacious than the expensive topical antibiotics which we used previously." The honey therapy reduced seven- to eight-week hospital stays by half.

By adding tea tree oil or grapefruit seed extract to raw honey, you can make a burn salve that is even more effective, for it will sterilize the wound on contact. I keep a squeeze bottle containing 5 ounces raw, unpasteurized honey mixed well with 1 ounce (2 tablespoons) tea tree oil and 1 teaspoon grapefruit seed extract on hand in the kitchen, and it's as effective in the treatment of cuts as it is for burns.

CANDIDIASIS (*CANDIDA ALBICANS*)

Who hasn't heard of Candida? Some call it the disease of the '80s, for that's when it became a popular diagnosis for anyone suffering from allergies, fatigue, chronic yeast infections, digestive problems, heartburn, intestinal bloating, mood swings, depression, PMS symptoms, insomnia, headaches, sinus problems, nagging coughs, numbness in the hands and legs, acne, kidney or bladder infections, arthritis, depression, canker sores and a host of other symptoms.

Candida albicans is a yeastlike fungus that grows in all of us. It inhabits the mouth, throat, intestines and genital tract, usually in healthy balance with bacteria and other yeasts. Candida overgrowth is what causes problems, and it often results from the use of antibiotics. Because these drugs kill beneficial as well as harmful bacteria, they allow Candida to flourish.

When Candida infects the mouth, it is called thrush. In the vagina, it results in vaginitis or yeast infections. Candida overgrowth in the intestines has been linked to food allergies or intolerances and other symptoms.

Both tea tree oil and grapefruit seed extract offer help to those plagued with candidiasis. Grapefruit seed extract taken orally (three or more capsules daily, or as directed by a health care professional) works from within to reduce Candida overgrowth, replacing more toxic antifungal drugs without disturbing friendly bacteria. Take debittered, dry grapefruit seed extract capsules or place 10 to 20 drops of liquid extract in an empty gelatin capsule just before swallowing.

Both grapefruit seed extract and tea tree oil make effective therapies for the bath, vaginal douching, toothbrush cleansing and mouth care.

Dr. Paul Belaiche studied the effect of essential oils that have antibacterial and antifungal properties, among them cinnamon oils from Ceylon and China, Spanish oregano, and savory from Provence, but all were highly irritating to vaginal mucous membranes. Noting that tea tree oil is far less irritating while having an antifungal action, he studied 28 women who suffered from vaginal candidiasis. Every night patients inserted a capsule containing a small amount of tea tree oil vaginally. Of the 28 patients, one discontinued treatment because of vaginal burning. At the end of 30 days, 23 patients were completely cured and their leucorrhea, a burning white discharge, had stopped. The remaining four continued treatment for a longer period and all showed improvement. Some medical practitioners who have followed Belaiche's lead prefer to have their patients saturate a tampon in a dilute solution of tea tree oil and leave it in place overnight, while others recommend douching with a few drops of tea tree oil diluted in water.

CHRONIC FATIGUE SYNDROME

Often associated with the Epstein-Barr virus, chronic fatigue syndrome brings a host of symptoms: fever, sore throat, swollen lymph nodes, extreme fatigue, loss of appetite, recurring respiratory infections, intestinal and digestive problems, jaundice, anxiety, depression, mood swings, irritability, sleep disturbances, sensitivity to heat and light, temporary memory loss, headache, loss of concentration, muscle spasms and aching joints. Like candidiasis, chronic fatigue syndrome resembles other illnesses and is not always diagnosed correctly. In fact, both diseases are often dismissed as psychiatric complaints.

Holistic health practitioners usually prescribe dietary improvements (fewer refined foods, more fresh vegetables and whole grains) and supplementation with vitamins and minerals, lecithin, acidophilus, proteolytic enzymes and essential fatty acids. Teas made from burdock root, dandelion, echinacea, goldenseal and pau d'arco are believed to be beneficial for those with chronic fatigue syndrome.

Because pathogens that enter the body in food or water pose a serious health risk to those with compromised immune systems, a growing number of health practitioners prescribe grapefruit seed extract as a support therapy. Take one or more capsules three times daily, or as prescribed by your health-care professional. To prevent any possible disruption of the balance of healthy intestinal flora during long-term treatment, consider alternating this therapy with other herbs or supplements every few weeks.

COLD SORES

Cold sores, also called fever blisters, are caused by the herpes simplex virus I. They develop under stress and the stress factors include infections, fevers, exposure to sun and wind, menstruation and anything that depresses the immune system. Cold sores are infectious, easily spread from one person to another or from one part of the body to another, and they don't respond to antibiotics. Creams and salves containing the amino acid lysine eliminate the virus, hence their widespread use in the treatment of cold sores. Both tea tree oil and grapefruit seed extract kill viruses on contact and they, too, are effective topical therapies. Apply full-strength or dilute tea tree oil or diluted grapefruit seed extract directly to the sore several times daily, as needed.

COLDS, FLU, SINUS INFECTIONS

Anyone who goes for two years without catching a cold or the flu in the U.S. has bragging rights. Our best-selling over-the-counter medications are our wealth of syrups, tablets, capsules and potions for the coughs, congestion, fever, sneezing, fatigue, headache and sore throats that accompany these illnesses.

One thing that really does help prevent colds and flu is a strong immune system. Chronic illnesses like candidiasis and chronic fatigue syndrome make a body vulnerable, so it makes sense to treat them. Taking grapefruit seed extract capsules daily during epidemics helps make you a less hospitable host to viruses and other pathogens, and if someone brings a cold or the flu to your home or place of business, common sense precautions include washing your hands frequently, spraying the air and door handles with an antiseptic solution of tea tree oil or grapefruit seed extract and sterilizing all exposed dishes, cups and eating utensils.

If you feel a chill in your bones, a sore throat, a fit of sneezing or a hacking cough, try to act as soon as the first symptoms appear. Take extra grapefruit seed extract and dose yourself frequently with tinctures or teas made of echinacea and other infection-fighting herbs, drink plenty of water and other liquids, and increase your vitamin C. Every hour or so rinse your mouth and gargle with a tea tree oil or grapefruit seed extract mouthwash, or simply add a few drops of either to a small amount of water to make your own. As often as possible, pour boiling water over a few drops of tea tree oil in a bowl, cover your head with a towel to make a tent, and breathe the resulting vapor. Keep your head well above the bowl to avoid scalding and breathe the vapor for as long as you can, for both the heat and the tea tree oil will help kill cold viruses. Apply a small amount of diluted tea tree oil directly to your nose, inside and out, to reinforce this effect. Rub full-strength or diluted tea tree oil onto the throat and chest, especially at bedtime.

To help relieve clogged nasal passages, use a nasal rinse. You can apply the rinse with a small glass instrument for nasal douching sold in pharmacies or use the long-nosed ceramic version sold in health food stores. Mix 2 ounces warm water with a pinch of sea salt and add 1 drop grape-fruit seed extract. Fill the applicator's reservoir, lean over the sink, close one nostril and let the water flow into the other. Slowly the water will work its way through sinus passages and begin to trickle through the other nostril. Repeat on the other side. Alternatively, pour the solution into your open palm and sniff it into nasal passages. A slightly salty solution is more soothing for mucous membranes and the grapefruit seed extract disinfects whatever it touches.

CRADLE CAP

An unsightly condition that coats the heads of tiny babies, cradle cap is the infant's form of adult dandruff. Tea tree oil has long been used to cure cradle cap. Mix 5 to 10 drops of tea tree oil in a small amount of olive oil (1 to 2 tea-spoons). Apply to the baby's scalp and massage gently. Let stand 5 minutes, then add a drop of tea tree oil to your baby's shampoo and wash well. Rinse with clear water.

CUTS

Superficial cuts, which include everything from paper cuts to injuries caused by the careless handling of kitchen knives, are easy to treat with nature's antiseptics. If you're near water and can rinse the wound, do so. Full-strength or dilute solutions of tea tree oil and grapefruit seed extract penetrate quickly through damaged tissue, and a coating of raw honey reduces pain by sealing the wound (see page 23). Bandage as appropriate, applying pressure with tape to hold the wound closed if necessary. Apply additional tea tree oil or grapefruit seed extract as needed.

In the case of deep puncture wounds or serious cuts that require stitching, seek medical attention.

CYSTITIS

Cystitis is a bladder infection caused by bacteria, usually *E. coli*, which is found in the intestines. Symptoms include an urgent need to urinate, painful or burning urination, a seeming inability to empty the bladder and the production of cloudy or unpleasant smelling urine.

Flushing the urinary tract is not the answer to cystitis; disinfection is. Cranberry juice, long a folk remedy for bladder infections, has performed well in clinical trials. Small quantities of unsweetened cranberry juice, available at health food stores, help prevent bacteria from thriving in the urinary tract. If the taste is too bitter, combine it with fruit juice. Uva ursi tea, often mislabeled as a diuretic, is an excellent urinary tract disinfectant and small, frequent doses of this astringent beverage speed healing. Grapefruit seed extract is another cystitis healer; take three or more capsules daily to help kill bacteria and reduce inflammation.

DANDRUFF

Although we call any flaking of the scalp dandruff, it may be caused by seborrhea, psoriasis, eczema or other infections. The topical application of either tea tree oil or grapefruit seed extract can cure any of these, restoring the scalp to its natural flake-free condition.

To treat any scalp condition, apply full-strength or diluted tea tree oil or diluted grapefruit seed extract directly to the scalp and massage well. Let stand several minutes, then shampoo hair. Alternatively, prepare a 5 percent to 10 percent solution of tea tree oil or grapefruit seed extract in olive oil (½ teaspoon extract in 2 tablespoons oil produces an 8 percent solution), massage into the scalp, cover hair with a shower cap and leave on overnight. In the morning, shampoo out.

To prevent a recurrence of dandruff, add several drops of tea tree oil or grapefruit seed extract to your shampoo or hair conditioner just before applying it, or mix 2 teaspoons oil or extract into 8 ounces of shampoo for a steady supply. Rinse thoroughly, and add a teaspoon of 15 percent solution to your final rinse water. In addition, consider that nutritional deficiencies are often linked to seborrheic dermatitis and other flaking conditions. Zinc, vitamins B2 and B6, biotin and essential fatty acids are often prescribed to improve this condition.

DERMATITIS

Sometimes called contact dermatitis or contact allergy, dermatitis is a scaling, itching rash or flaking skin condition caused by exposure to metal alloys (nickel in jewelry is a common source), perfumes, cosmetics, latex, medicated lotions or toxic plants like poison oak and ivy.

For most dermatitis, a dilute solution of tea tree oil or an antiseptic cream containing tea tree oil helps alleviate itching, swelling and redness. Apply frequently. In cases of poison oak or ivy, tea tree oil helps dissolve and remove the plant resins that cause the irritation. Grapefruit seed extract treats the rashes of contact dermatitis, including poison oak and ivy, as well.

DIAPER RASH

Diaper rash is usually caused by yeasts such as *Candida albicans*. Conventional treatment consists of medicated salves and powders and, in severe cases, the ingestion of antifungal drugs such as Nystatin. A natural alternative is the application of dilute tea tree oil or grapefruit seed extract, or a salve or lotion containing either, supplemented by grapefruit seed extract taken orally. Instead of administering a powerful drug that has potential side effects and which destroys friendly bacteria, a capsule of powdered, debittered grapefruit seed extract can be opened and mixed with milk or food. The dosage should be determined by an experienced health professional, but one capsule (equivalent to 10 to 15 drops of concentrate) divided into several portions and administered over a two-day period is a conservative starting point and the dosage can be increased as required. Acidophilus supplementation or live culture yogurt will be helpful as well. If the mother is breast-feeding, whatever she eats or drinks will be transferred to her baby, and she can take three or more capsules of grapefruit seed extract in addition to live acidophilus supplements daily.

Add a few drops of water-soluble tea tree oil concentrate or grapefruit seed extract to the baby's bath water, wipe the baby well with dilute tea tree oil or grapefruit seed extract at every diaper changing and replace his or her baby oil with a blend of olive oil (or another carrier oil) and grapefruit seed extract or tea tree oil. *Never apply full-strength tea tree oil or grapefruit seed extract to a baby's skin; always dilute it with water or a carrier oil first.*

DIARRHEA

Diarrhea isn't always caused by food or water contamination, parasites or bacteria, but these are common sources. Grapefruit seed extract is probably best known for its ability to prevent traveler's diarrhea, whether it's caused by *Giardia lamblia*, the tiny parasite that infects North America's lakes, or by unfamiliar bacteria we encounter in foreign countries. As literature from ProSeed grapefruit seed extract explains:

> Although there's no substitute for common sense, taking grapefruit seed liquid extract or capsules internally every day as directed (starting a few days before your trip) will help you stay well and feel great while experiencing exotic locales your friends only dream about. Place a few drops in a glass of water, stir well, and a few seconds later the water is free from a wide variety of microbes, fungi, viruses, parasites and bacteria. If your food is contaminated, drinking the grapefruit seed extract activated water should help protect you against diarrhea and other maladies. (Obviously, if you know it's contaminated, tactfully refrain from indulging.) It could well protect you against staphylococcus, streptococcus, salmonella and a multitude of viruses and fungi now widespread globally. Although no product

could possibly guarantee 100% success, this liquid will significantly reduce your traveling risks.

The recommended dose is one capsule three times daily, or 10 to 15 drops liquid extract taken in juice or by capsule, or as prescribed by a health care professional. The same dosage will treat active cases of diarrhea.

DOG BITES

The first thing to do with any dog, cat or other animal bite is disinfect it, and the easiest way to treat a broken skin injury is with a dilute solution of tea tree oil or grapefruit seed extract. Both are powerful antiseptics and they will destroy on contact nearly every bacteria or pathogen they touch. Flush the bite with dilute tea tree oil or grapefruit seed extract, then cleanse the area with soap and water and apply more antiseptic solution. Repeat applications of full-strength tea tree oil or a dilute solution of tea tree oil or grapefruit seed extract three times daily for several days. Obviously, if the bite is serious or if you have no way of verifying the dog's rabies vaccination, it is important to seek medical attention.

EAR INFECTIONS

More than any other condition, chronic ear infections are the reason American children take so many antibiotics. While antibiotics are powerful drugs with significant side effects, they don't provide a lasting cure. Typically, ear infections recur and with each reinfection, the drugs are less effective.

Both tea tree oil and grapefruit seed extract are proven ear infection fighters. The simplest approach is to apply several drops of diluted tea tree oil or grapefruit seed extract solution into each ear or saturate a cotton ball and hold it against the ear orifice several times a day until the infection clears. ProSeed makes an ear drop product that contains extracts of plantain and mullein, two appropriate healing herbs, in a vegetable glycerine base. Wherever mullein grows, herbalists gather its yellow blossoms to make a mullein and olive oil infusion renowned as a cure for ear infections. You can buy mullein oil (not to be confused with an essential oil made by distillation) in health food stores or herbal tea shops, where it is often labeled mullein ear oil or something similar, and add several drops of tea tree oil and/or grapefruit seed extract for faster action. The advantage to using vegetable glycerine or olive oil as a carrier for tea tree oil or grapefruit seed extract is that they are sticky and tend to stay in place. Whatever product you decide to use, place its glass eyedropper bottle in hot water until the contents are warm to the touch. Warm ear drops are especially soothing.

Children aren't the only ones who get ear infections. Adults do, too, and so do pets. Swimmer's ear, which afflicts children and teenagers, especially during the summer, is an outer ear infection caused by water-borne viruses, bacteria, fungi, parasites and other pathogens; its symptoms include a feeling of fullness in the ear, excessive wax, irritation and itching, but acute infections bring pain and discharge as well. Water dogs with floppy ears, like Labrador retrievers, have their own version of swimmer's ear. All of the treatments described here are effective in treating swimmer's ear and other ear infections in both pets and people.

FUNGAL INFECTIONS

Athlete's foot, jock itch, toenail fungus and ringworm are only four of the fungal infections that annoy, itch, disfigure and irritate human beings, some of them lasting for years. Tea tree oil and grapefruit seed extract kill fungi on contact, and both have proven track records in the treatment of these unpleasant conditions.

In most cases grapefruit seed extract is diluted before application, but in the case of nail fungus it can be dropped full strength on affected toenails and fingernails. Do the same with full-strength tea tree oil. Massage well into surrounding tissue and be sure to saturate all sides of the nail surface.

Jock itch, athlete's foot and nail fungus thrive in warm, damp, dark conditions. In addition to applying full-strength or diluted tea tree oil or grapefruit seed extract, soaking affected feet in footbaths containing their solutions, drying skin surfaces well with absorbent toweling or a hair dryer, powdering the skin well to keep it dry and wearing socks, shoes and underwear that breathe and keep moisture away from the skin, you can take grapefruit seed extract internally to speed healing and make your system more resistant to fungal infections.

GUM DISEASE

Periodontal disease. Receding gums. Gingivitis. Pyorrhea. Bleeding gums. Abscesses. Gum surgery. Ouch!

Periodontal means "around a tooth" and it refers to any disorder of the gums and mouth. Gingivitis is an inflammation of the gums considered to be an early stage of pyorrhea, which is also called periodontitis. The causes of these unpleasant maladies are bacteria, mucus, the accumulation of plaque, poor nutrition, improper brushing, serious illnesses, smoking, drug use and excessive alcohol.

Two of the best gum and tooth protectors are tea tree oil and grapefruit seed extract. Product catalogs abound with special mouth care products made from these natural antiseptics: toothpastes, mouthwashes, dental floss, breath-freshening mouth drops, lozenges, gum cleansers and toothpicks. You can buy these special products or make your own by adding tea tree oil or grapefruit seed extract to whatever you already use.

If you have bleeding gums, an abscess, inflammation or infection anywhere in your mouth, try applying full-strength tea tree oil several times a day, or rinse your mouth with a dilute solution of tea tree oil or grapefruit seed extract, holding the solution in your mouth for as long as possible before spitting it out. These are not the most pleasant-tasting products, but their effects are dramatic. To make the treatment more palatable, follow the instructions on page 46 for adding flavor oils.

No matter what type of toothbrush you use, keep it germ-free by soaking the brush in a dilute solution of tea tree oil or grapefruit seed extract (5 to 10 drops in ½ cup water) for

10 minutes, then rinse. If you use a Water Pik or similar device, add a few drops to the water reservoir whenever you use it.

In Australia, it is not uncommon for dentists to use tea tree oil in the treatment of tooth decay, adding it directly to cavities before and after drilling for fillings, saturating tooth sockets after extractions, and instructing their patients to apply it to diseased teeth for several days before drilling or extraction to reduce complications. The most common complication of modern dentistry is infection, and tea tree oil has an impressive record of preventing infections in the mouth. The dental journal *Periodontology* published a study designed to confirm or disprove reports of tea tree oil's antimicrobial effects on the organisms associated with tooth decay. The researchers found that full-strength, undiluted tea tree oil has the greatest antimicrobial activity and that it has significant action against oral pathogens.

HALITOSIS

Bad breath or halitosis can result from eating garlic and other odoriferous foods, in which case the unpleasant effect disappears in a day or two, but chronic bad breath is often a byproduct of gum disease or tooth decay. Regular use of tea tree oil or grapefruit seed extract as described in the preceding section will improve halitosis.

HEAD LICE

Head lice are in the headlines. Throughout the 1990s, public and private schools have been sending students home because of head lice epidemics. One reason for the problem's sudden severity, according to public health officials, is that lice are becoming resistant to the drugs that have controlled them in the past. Not only are most of these drugs highly toxic (Greenpeace and other ecology organizations warn that even tiny amounts in lakes or rivers can cause major fish kills) but they have potentially adverse side effects in children.

Head lice spread quickly from one person to another, either through personal contact or on shared combs, brushes and other objects. Lice lay their eggs on hair shafts and then burrow into the scalp, where their excrement causes intense itching. Scratching the head deposits eggs under fingernails, which is why the creatures spread so quickly. Everything an infected person touches is contaminated.

The simplest cure for head lice in those who have short hair is daily shampooing and blow drying. The heat from a blow dryer is often sufficient to destroy both the mites and their eggs, which is why when a family becomes infected, it is often the father who suffers least.

Tea tree oil is a powerful solvent, and it is said to dissolve lice eggs on contact. No matter how it works, tea tree oil is a very effective delouser.

To treat a louse infestation, use either of the following therapies.

Apply full-strength tea tree oil or water-soluble tea tree oil concentrate to the head and scalp. Massage well so that it is evenly distributed and all hair shafts are coated. If your hair is very long, you may need more. Cover the hair with a shower cap or hot towel and let stand for 10 to 15 minutes. Shampoo thoroughly and rinse. Repeat this treatment after 48 hours.

Alternatively, wash with a solution of 3 tablespoons shampoo plus 2 tablespoons full-strength tea tree oil. Apply the lather to the head and entire body and let it stand for three to five minutes. Rinse well, use any leftover shampoo to give your hair another sudsing and rinse again. Add 1 tablespoon water-soluble tea tree oil concentrate to a plastic pitcher of hot water for the final rinse. Some practitioners recommend adding a tablespoon of apple cider vinegar to this rinse.

Lice don't just live on people's heads, they thrive wherever there's body hair. When lice infect the pubic area, they are called crabs.

To avoid recontamination, be sure to wash all bed linens, towels and recently used clothing in hot water, adding tea tree oil to the wash water, and dry in a hot dryer. Disinfect combs, brushes, eyebrow brushes and other grooming tools in hot water containing tea tree oil. Don't loan or borrow these items, and wash your hands frequently, especially in schools and other crowded public places.

HERPES (GENITAL HERPES)

The herpes virus causes several illnesses, including chicken pox, cold sores and shingles. But its most painful affliction may be genital herpes, which attacks the genitals with itching, reddened skin that erupts into small painful blisters. Genital herpes is sexually transmitted, highly infectious and, worst of all, recurring. Herpes attacks, which are precipitated by stress, are usually worse in women than men, and pregnant women are at special risk because they can transmit the virus and its complications, which include brain damage and blindness, to their babies.

Because genital herpes is caused by a virus, it does not respond to antibiotics and there is no known cure. Orthodox treatment includes oral drugs and topical ointments designed to alleviate pain, prevent outbreaks and keep the virus from spreading.

Tea tree oil, which requires no prescription and which has no adverse side effects, penetrates deeply into infected tissue, kills the herpes virus and alleviates inflammation and itching, making this simple remedy an effective treatment for herpes outbreaks. It is helpful to add tea tree oil to bath water and to spray affected areas with a dilute solution. Like tea tree oil, grapefruit seed extract is a powerful antiviral agent and it, too, can be applied in dilute solution to herpes outbreaks. Taking grapefruit seed extract internally may also speed healing and help prevent outbreaks from recurring.

HOUSEHOLD USE

Both tea tree oil and grapefruit seed extract have so many household uses, it's impossible to list them all. Here are a few applications:

• To disinfect kitchen surfaces, telephone receivers, door knobs and even the air around you, spray with a dilute solution of either product. Add tea tree oil or grapefruit seed extract to liquid hand soap as described on page 44.

• To disinfect meat, poultry, eggs, fish, fruit and vegetables, fill a sink with cold water and add 15 to 30 drops of grapefruit seed extract and soak for a few minutes, then rinse. (Soak produce items separately from meat items.) Disinfect food items while washing by spraying them first with a dilute solution.

• To disinfect laundry and control mold and odors, add 20 to 40 drops full-strength grapefruit seed extract or water-soluble tea tree oil concentrate to wash water. Add a smaller amount to your kitchen or bathroom floor's wash water before mopping. Control mold and odors on bathroom walls, shower curtains and shower doors by applying a dilute solution of tea tree oil or grapefruit seed extract with a sponge.

• Disinfect air conditioner units, humidifiers and the collection pans of dehumidifiers with either solution. It can be sprayed into air ducts and onto filters; a few drops will disinfect humidifiers, vaporizers and dehumidifiers.

INSECT BITES, STINGS AND WOUNDS

One of the most dramatic stories told about tea tree oil's healing powers was reported by Harry Bungwahl of New South Wales to the Thursday Plantation tea tree oil company. Bungwahl was bitten on the foot by a funnel-web spider, notorious as one of the world's most dangerous arachnids. Occasionally fatal and always extremely painful, funnel-web spider bites require immediate medical attention. The victim's wife phoned the local hospital while he applied tea tree oil to the wound. By the time he reached the hospital his foot had stopped hurting, though his lips and fingers were still tingling. Hospital staff confirmed the spider's identification. Bungwahl was given no medical treatment but was kept under observation for four hours and then discharged. He suffered no ill effects from the bite and was most impressed with tea tree oil's alleviation of its pain.

Those familiar with tea tree oil consider it an antidote and treatment for all venomous bites, stings and wounds.

Immediate application of tea tree oil neutralizes wasp, bee, centipede, fire ant and spider venom and it stops the itch and swelling of flea and mosquito bites. It is believed to help neutralize more potent venoms, such as those from snake and scorpion bites, if applied in time.

At the first sign of a bite, apply full-strength tea tree oil, not once but several times. Saturate the area well and give the oil every opportunity to penetrate deep into the affected area. Pain and itching should stop within minutes. If the bite is serious, seek medical attention, but apply your tea tree oil first.

Like tea tree oil, grapefruit seed extract is a powerful anti-microbial. It will destroy bacteria, viruses and other pathogens on contact. Full-strength or slightly diluted grapefruit seed extract will quickly disinfect any bite.

Several books and articles about tea tree oil recommend applying the oil to ticks that are still attached to the bodies of people or their pets. This is supposed to kill the tick so that it drops off harmlessly. However, the Lyme disease authorities I interviewed cautioned against this approach because applying external agents to a still-attached tick causes an involuntary muscular contraction in the tick, which empties the contents of its digestive tract through the bite, like a hypodermic injection. Instead of using tea tree oil to kill the tick, they suggest removing the tick with tweezers, then immediately applying either full-strength tea tree oil, 3 percent hydrogen peroxide or both. The topical disinfectant hydrogen peroxide, sold in drug stores, kills Lyme disease bacteria, for these spirochetes are anaerobic and cannot survive in an oxygen-rich environment.

Last, anyone who climbs around tropical swamps should know that tea tree oil is toxic to leeches. Apply a drop to a biting leech and it will let go and fall off. Add another drop or two to the bite.

INSECT REPELLANT

Most of us would love to find a safe, nontoxic, effective insect repellant. Health food stores offer several, usually based on citronella and pennyroyal. Others combine more exotic ingredients. Do they work?

Yes and no. Herbal insect repellants have to be applied far more often than their chemical counterparts, and each type seems to be more effective for some people than others. You will have to experiment with yourself and your local insect population to find the right combination, but the effort is well worthwhile.

In the June/July 1994 issue of *The Herb Companion*, Arthur O. Tucker reviewed the scientific literature on herbs and insects. Mosquitoes are the most thoroughly examined insects, and in various studies, the essential oils of citronella, basil and juniper have been shown to repel them. In preliminary testing, rose geranium, rosemary and several species of cedar have also shown promise. Citronella, palmarosa, juniper and rose geranium repel the common housefly and some evidence suggests that sweet flag root, Kenyan myrrh, bog myrtle, German chamomile, sandalwood and vetiver may as well.

For fleas, pennyroyal is the perennial favorite, but note that full-strength pennyroyal oil is highly toxic and has contributed to the deaths of several household pets, even when used as directed in small doses. Always dilute pennyroyal oil. Lemon oil is fatal to cat fleas and is sold as a "natural" flea dip, but while citrus oils are indeed natural, they are highly toxic to cats. If you use these oils as flea repellants, apply them to your pet's bedding instead of the animal itself. Well-diluted pennyroyal and lemon oils can be used in repellant sprays. Other reported flea repellants include California laurel and the leaves and branches of black walnut trees.

Because of Lyme disease and Rocky Mountain spotted fever, everyone wants to find a tick repellant that works. In his article, Tucker cited evidence that opopanax or bisabol myrrh (*Commiphora erythraea*), which is the myrrh of ancient Egypt, kills tick larvae on contact and repels adult African brown ear ticks, dog ticks and Lone Star ticks. He speculated that the essential oil of common myrrh (*C. myrrha*), which is more readily available, might do the same. Other herbs cited in the scientific literature as having tick-repelling properties include rose geranium, rosemary and California laurel.

Barbara Hall, a New York herbalist who is an expert on Lyme disease, decided to test African myrrh, rose geranium oil, rosemary oil and laurel tincture on live ticks donated by her cat. She was especially interested in deer ticks, now called black-legged ticks, which are most associated with Lyme disease. Only rose-scented geranium repelled the ticks, and Hall created a simple, effective recipe: combine 20 drops rose geranium essential oil, 3 drops citronella oil and a splash of bay leaf tincture in 10 ounces of water. Rose geranium keeps the ticks away, the citronella repels flies and mosquitoes, and bay leaf adds a pleasant fragrance.

Although they are widely reputed to repel mosquitoes, flies and other insects, lemon grass and eucalyptus have repeatedly been shown to be ineffective. And even though fans of tea tree oil claim it is a natural insect repellant, my experiments with full-strength and diluted tea tree oil on ticks, black flies and mosquitoes have been only partly successful. For the record, Cynthia Olsen claims in her book *Australian Tea Tree Oil Guide* that tea tree oil is an excellent flea repellant. I enjoy the oil's antiseptic fragrance and appreciate its skin-soothing benefits, so my herbal insect repellant consists of 1 tablespoon bay rum tincture (see instructions on page 44), ½ teaspoon tea tree oil, 25 drops rose geranium oil and 5 drops citronella oil, mixed well to dissolve the essential oils and make them water soluble, plus 16 ounces (1 pint) water.

MUSCLE ACHES, PAINS

With its analgesic benefits and deep penetration, tea tree oil is an effective therapy for sports injuries and strained muscles. It can be applied full strength, as a dilute solution or added to massage oils. To help protect specific muscles, apply the tea tree oil before engaging in vigorous activity as well as after. Adding tea tree oil to bath water is also therapeutic.

PET CARE

Dogs and cats are more than animals, they're members of the family. So are our birds, hamsters, guinea pigs and a host of other creatures.

Hair and coat problems are probably the most common complaints among dog and cat owners, next to flea infestations. It is easier to prevent fleas than to remove them once established, but frequent vacuuming, careful grooming with a fine toothed flea comb (which removes adult fleas and eggs along with shed fur), washing pet bedding and similar items in very hot water, bathing pets with tea tree oil shampoo and spraying the area with flea repellent herbal oils (see *Insect Repellants*) will help remove even well-established fleas. Improving your pet's diet is another important step, for fleas are less attracted to healthy dogs and cats.

You'll find a variety of herbal sprays containing tea tree oil in pet supply stores as well as health food stores for use on dogs and cats. These sprays treat hot spots, allergic dermatitis and other skin irritations. Their companion products, herbal shampoos and conditioners, help improve a coat's appearance.

Both tea tree oil and grapefruit seed extract can be added to pet shampoos, rinses and herbal sprays. Both combat viruses, bacteria, fungi, yeasts, mold and other pathogens. Their dilute solutions can be applied to ringworm, infected wounds, eczema, flea bites, fungal lesions, pustules, rashes, bare spots and sores.

Because parasites are such a serious problem, grapefruit seed extract capsules can be given to dogs and cats to help prevent worms. The capsules contain debittered, powdered extract, which can be sprinkled over food. Dogs weighing 50 lbs. or more can take two or three capsules daily, or as recommended by a holistic veterinarian; smaller dogs can start with a single capsule or half of one.

All of these therapies, diluted or adjusted for the animal's size and species, can be used on other animals.

Note: Never use full-strength tea tree oil or grapefruit seed extract on your pet. Always dilute these products first. Because the taste of tea tree oil is so unpleasant, some herbalists recommend its application on body parts that an animal chews or licks incessantly, such as its leg or tail. However, the September 1994 issue of the veterinary journal *Small Animal Medicine and Surgery* warns, "*Melaleuca toxicosis* has been reported to the National Animal Poison Control Center when the oil has been applied topically in appropriately high doses to treat dermatological conditions in dogs and cats." Symptoms, which occurred within two to eight hours of application, included depression, weakness, incoordination and muscle tremors. The reaction disappeared within three to four days. Even when you use a 15 percent solution of tea tree oil or grapefruit seed extract on your dog or cat, be careful to avoid the eye area, watch the animal carefully for adverse symptoms and, if they occur, discontinue use.

PSORIASIS AND ECZEMA

Psoriasis and eczema are only two of the troublesome skin diseases that cause inflammation, flaking, lesions and unsightly rashes. They are treated with an assortment of drugs, all of which are effective to some degree and none of which are called a cure.

Holistic physicians approach these illnesses through nutrition, improving the diet and prescribing supplements while checking for food sensitivities. Both tea tree oil and grapefruit seed extract can be applied to affected areas (always dilute grapefruit seed extract) and grapefruit seed capsules can be taken at the same time. Salves and ointments containing these natural antiseptics help soften and repair skin while fighting the infection. For best results, apply dilute tea tree oil or grapefruit seed extract to dry skin, then follow with a salve, ointment or lotion. Repeat as desired.

SCABIES

A tiny mite causes scabies, which is an infectious skin disease spread by contact with infected people or inanimate materials like bedding. The mite burrows into the skin and lays eggs, which hatch and cause all kinds of discomfort.

Most often scabies attack the skin between fingers, the fingers themselves, palms, wrists and genital areas. Inflammation and intense itching are its major symptoms.

The orthodox treatment of scabies is the same as for lice: the application of pesticides. Tea tree oil works just as well, and its anti-inflammatory properties give immediate relief of itching and swelling. Dilute solutions of tea tree oil are as effective as full-strength tea tree oil in destroying the scabies mite and its eggs. Apply several times a day for two days, then as desired.

SUNBURN

Sunburn, like any scald or burn, inflames the skin, causes pain and swelling, damages skin and promotes infection.

To treat sunburn, dilute water-soluble tea tree oil concentrate in a strong chamomile tea, comfrey tea or aloe vera gel. All of these are skin healers; chamomile reduces inflammation, comfrey contains a powerful cell growth stimulant and aloe vera soothes and heals burned skin. Alternatively, apply full-strength or diluted tea tree oil to burned areas. Tea tree oil penetrates quickly through damaged layers, reducing pain and swelling and preventing infection.

WARTS

Warts are caused by a virus, and both tea tree oil and grapefruit seed extracts kill viruses. Any wart, whether a common wart on the hands or face, genital warts or plantar warts on the feet, can be treated with full-strength or dilute tea tree oil or a dilute solution of grapefruit seed extract. Apply three times daily, using enough to saturate the wart and surrounding tissue.

IMPROVING ON PERSONAL CARE PRODUCTS

DISINFECTANT SOAP

If you use liquid hand soap in pump dispensers, add 2 teaspoons of tea tree oil or grapefruit seed extract to 12 ounces liquid soap and stir to mix well. It isn't necessary to buy expensive antibacterial soaps; a gentle olive oil–based liquid soap from the health food store with added tea tree oil or grapefruit seed extract will be kinder to hands and just as antiseptic. If you prefer bar soap, use a tea tree oil soap or add a drop of tea tree oil or grapefruit seed extract to your soap's lather while washing.

HAIR CARE

To any shampoo, hair conditioner or hair care product, add several drops of tea tree oil or grapefruit seed extract. Massage well into scalp before rinsing to reduce dandruff and improve the scalp.

FRAGRANT LOTIONS

If you like the smell of bay rum, try making your own bay rum aftershave. It's better than anything you can buy because it contains no synthetic ingredients—nothing but the best! To prepare bay rum extract, buy fresh or dried bay leaves at the supermarket. Fill a small glass jar with leaves loosely packed and cover with high proof or regular rum. Tighten cap. Leave in a warm, dark place for several weeks, shaking occasionally. You are creating a tincture, which is an alcohol extract. The longer it stands, the stronger the bay rum fragrance. For an even more concentrated tincture, prepare a second jar of fresh or dried bay leaves and, after three or four weeks of tincturing, pour the rum solution over the new bay leaves and repeat the process.

Mix 1 ounce (2 tablespoons) full-strength tea tree oil with enough strained bay rum tincture (start with 2 ounces or 4 tablespoons) to make the oil water soluble. Shake the combination in a small glass jar or plastic bottle and let it stand for a few minutes. If there is an oily film on the surface or if you see drops of oil, add more tincture. If desired, add a tablespoon of vegetable glycerine to the solution for a more soothing, emollient lotion.

Test the result on your skin. This solution can be used as is, or you can dilute it with water to make a thinner lotion. It is appropriate for both men and women and will help heal cuts or scrapes even in delicate areas, like along the bikini line. It can be applied after waxing or other methods of hair removal.

Men who are prone to ingrown hairs can help prevent them by lightly dry brushing the face with a loofah or buffing sponge before shaving, then saturating the skin with tea tree oil lotion. Women can prevent ingrown hairs on the legs by dry brushing with a loofah or Japanese vegetable bristle bath brush and applying the lotion.

Try other essential oils and tinctures, too. For example, instead of making bay rum, make a tincture of lavender blossoms, rosemary, sage or a combination of favorite herbs. To the tea tree oil, add a few drops of cinnamon oil or other essential oils. Substitute grapefruit seed extract for all or part of the tea tree oil. There is no limit to the fragrant lotions you can create and all of them will be therapeutic and antiseptic.

DEODORANT

Tea tree oil makes an effective deodorant, by itself or in combination with other essential oils. To make your own deodorant spray, combine tea tree oil with a few drops of grapefruit seed extract, an essential oil such as lavender, lemon, bayberry or sage, enough alcohol or bay rum tincture to dissolve the oils, a dollop of vegetable glycerine and enough water to form a pleasing solution. Spray under arms, on feet or wherever needed.

TOOTH AND MOUTH CARE

Add a drop of tea tree oil or grapefruit seed extract to the toothpaste on your brush. Massage full-strength or diluted tea tree oil onto gums. Add a drop or two of tea tree oil or grapefruit seed extract to a small amount of mouthwash before rinsing. Make your own mouthwash by adding 10 to 15 drops of the essential oil of cinnamon, cloves, nutmeg or ginger, or any combination of these spices, to your water-soluble tea tree oil concentrate or to a teaspoon of grapefruit seed extract, then dilute with water to the desired strength. Or, instead of diluting this solution for use as a mouthwash, leave it more concentrated and apply a few drops to your toothbrush when you brush your teeth, massaging your gums well, or apply it with a fingertip. Soak toothpicks or Stim-U-Dents in the concentrated solution, then let them dry for more flavorful gum stimulation. Dip dental floss in the solution before using. Use it to disinfect toothbrushes. Tea tree oil and grapefruit seed extract can be your mouth's best friends.

RESOURCES

MANUFACTURERS AND DISTRIBUTORS

For more about tea tree oil, contact the following companies:

Desert Essence, 9510 Vasser Avenue, Unit A, Chatsworth, CA 91311, phone (818) 709-4900.

Thursday Plantation, Inc., 330 East Carrillo Street, Santa Barbara, CA 93101, phone 1-800-848-8966.

For information about grapefruit seed extract and products containing it, contact:

Imhotep, Inc. (ProSeed), PO Box 183, Ruby, NY 12475, phone 1-800-677-8577.

NutriBiotic (Citricidal), 865 Parallel Drive, Lakeport, CA 95453, phone (707) 263-1475.

Allergy Research Group (Nutricology, Paramicrocidin), 22 N. Vincent Avenue, Covina, CA 91722, phone (510) 639-4572.

TEA TREE OIL LABELS

In the United States, it is not necessary to identify a product as synthetic rather than natural, and some firms use synthetic tea tree oil, which does not contain the complex organic compounds of natural oil and is less effective. Some products contain species other than *Melaleuca alternifolia* and are adulterations. To be sure your oil meets the Australian standard, look for these claims on the label: 100 percent tea tree oil, *Melaleuca alternifolia* and product of Australia.

HERBAL PRODUCTS, INFORMATION SOURCES

Herbal products and essential oils can be purchased from most health food stores, herbal tea companies and herb supply shops. For a free mail order catalog of herbs and herbal supplies, contact Jean's Greens, 54 McMannus Road, Rensselaerville, NY 12147.

For information about herbs and herbalists, contact the Northeast Herbal Association, PO Box 479, Milton, NY 12547; the Herb Research Foundation, 1007 Pearl Street, Suite 200, Boulder, CO 80302, phone 1-800-748-2617; and the American Herbal Association, PO Box 1673, Nevada City, CA 95959.

Recommended reading: *The Herb Quarterly*, Long Mountain Press, 223 San Anselmo Avenue, Suite 7, San Anselmo,

CA 94960, and *The Herb Companion*, Interweave Press, 201 East Fourth Street, Loveland, CO 80537.

BIBLIOGRAPHY

Brouse, Richard. *Melaleuca: Nature's Antiseptic.* Clackamas, Oregon: Sunnyside Health Center, 1989.

Drury, Susan. *Tea Tree Oil: A Medicine Kit in a Bottle.* Saffron Walden, Essex, England: C.W. Daniel Company, Ltd., 1991.

Foster, Stephen. "Tea Tree and Its Relatives: A Little Medicine, a Little Marketing." *The Herb Companion*, February/March 1994, pages 48–51.

————. "Why the To-Do about Tea Tree Oil?" *Vegetarian Times*, October 1995, pages 98–101.

Igram, Cass. *Killed on Contact: The Tea Tree Oil Story, Nature's Finest Antiseptic.* Cedar Rapids, Iowa: Literary Visions Publishing, 1992.

Lawless, Julia. *The Encyclopedia of Essential Oils.* Rockport, Massachusetts: Element, Inc., 1992.

Metcalfe, Joannah. *Herbs and Aromatherapy.* New York: Seafarer Books, 1994.

Olsen, Cynthia B. *Australian Tea Tree Oil First Aid Handbook.* Pegosa Spring, Colorado: Kali Press, 1991.

————. *Australian Tea Tree Oil Guide.* Pegosa Spring, Colorado: Kali Press, 1991.

————. "Australian Tea Tree Oil: Nature's Wonder from Down Under." *Health World*, August 1992, pages 44–45.

Winters, Sir Jason. *Breakthrough: In Search of an Australian Legend, Miracle Healing Oil of the Ages.* Las Vegas: Vinton Publishing, 1986.